MW01520446

Do you still have cleavage with just one breast?

Just married
and newly pregnant
Sue finds a lump
in her breast.
This is her
intimate diary.

Sue Lawrence PhD

First Edition 2016

First Published in the United Kingdom by Springtime Books

Design: Leigh Cann, lcann563@gmail.com

Cover design: Leigh Cann

ISBN: 978-0-9932377-5-1

To Sheila – a warrior!

With love + best

wishes,

Sue.

To Elona – my why

ACKNOWLEDGEMENTS

I really appreciated everyone's kindness and support. First, I'd like to thank Kristof and Marianne. Thank you to thank my Canadian family – Joyce, Sandra, Gerald, Frank, John, Clare, Kayley and Kendra, and my Belgium family – Jan, Mimi, Stefan, Katrien, Celéste and Jule for their support and kindness throughout our cancer journey.

A big thank you goes to my friends Susan Allan, Emma Bassemann, Joke Cornelius, Tena Ganovichef, Ingrid Hu, Suzie Gilles, Sherrill Johnson, Donna King, Jolene Skordis-Worrall and Laura Shipler-Chico for providing good times and support.

Thanks to my new Delft friends, Jasmina Campochiaro, Manuela Damant, Helga Kristina Fridjonsdottir, Ana Luz, Anna Molinari, Judit Rapai, Colleen Reichrath-Smith and Jennifer Soerohardjo who made this book and the Nipple Party possible.

Thanks to my PhD supervisor and friend Professor Antonia Bifulco for her patience and support. And finally, a hearty thank you to Jo Parfitt for saying "yes".

TABLE OF CONTENTS

PHOTOGRAPHS

Photo 1:   Kristof and Sue's Wedding Day.

Photo 2:   Elona and I in the Misericordia
             Hospital, Edmonton, Canada. Elona
             is a few days old

Photo 3:   Elona under the blue light – a few
             hours old.

Photo 4:   Kristof, the proud papa.

Photo 5:   Elona and I after my first run
             (Elona is six months old).

Photo 6:   Elona is sunshine (three and a half
             years old).

Photo 7:   The Champagne Shimmy at My Nipple
             Party, Hotel Vermeer, Delft.

Photo 8:   Alma Boerland presented me with my
             Nipple on a chocolate heart.

FOREWORDS

Sometimes we make a new friendship in the unlikeliest of places. I met Sue Lawrence for the first time on April 8, 2008, in the chemotherapy room at the Cross Cancer Institute in Edmonton, Alberta, Canada. She was at the beginning of her journey with breast cancer while I was in my eighth year of ongoing maintenance treatment. Our connection was immediate despite the thirty-year age difference. Our discussion was open and frank. We talked about the ups and downs, the joys and sorrows, the hope and despair, the messiness of dealing with a breast cancer diagnosis. The emotional havoc it wreaked on our relationships. No aspect was off limits. Thus began a deep friendship, which continues to this day.

An avid writer, Sue kept a diary of her journey, excerpts from which form the basis of this book – a raw, emotional and brutally honest account. Living with cancer is a daily battle emotionally, physically and mentally. It can also be lonely. Our friends and family often don't 'get it'. As Sue says, they talk about the end of the race before we've even come out of the starting blocks. Sue spares nothing in her account. She is unflinching in describing her daily struggles and innermost feelings. Anyone living with cancer will recognize themselves in these pages. Each journey is both unique and universal. Sue's rage, anxieties, self-doubt, determination and hopefulness will resonate with the reader. Friends and family will gain insight into the type of support their loved one needs. Early in our friendship I began to refer to Sue as a Warrior Queen. Her journey has been particularly turbulent. Diagnosed with breast cancer in her third month of pregnancy she underwent a mastectomy, later discovering she had the BRCA II gene and had a second mastectomy – followed by breast reconstruction – and in 2012 still more surgery to have her fallopian tubes removed. This was surely enough turmoil to make anyone cave in, yet Sue stood her battleground. Not always with ease though. Even a Warrior Queen must occasionally lay down her battle sword to lick her wounds and shed some tears before she can regroup for the next charge.

A cancer diagnosis is life altering. There is no one, right way to navigate its tumultuous waters. Sue has courageously shared her odyssey in the hope that others on a similar journey will draw comfort and reassurance from her story and feel less alone: that they will give themselves permission to acknowledge and express the myriad emotions which accompany diagnosis and treatment; that their family and friends will listen without judgment and without uttering idle platitudes.

Thankfully my Warrior Queen has laid down her sword but she still stands on guard. My hope is that this book is only the first instalment of many chapters to come.

Marianne McInnes
October 2015

After my sister, Sue, was diagnosed with breast cancer, I started to look at our family history and began to wonder if we should be looking into genetic testing. Our cousin Brenda had recently been treated for breast cancer and our Aunt Lily died of ovarian cancer years earlier. I asked my doctor for a mammogram soon after Sue's diagnosis. I was told I didn't need to worry because at 44, I was too young for a mammogram. But I persisted. In the end, they gave in and I had the mammogram in December 2007.To my great relief there were no tumours and all appeared well. However, my requests for genetic testing did not have the same positive results. There was no referral to the Genetics Department so I put this quest aside and focused on supporting my sister.

We were all shocked with her diagnosis. "How could this happen?" we kept asking ourselves. After the joy of her wedding and the revelation she was pregnant, now this? So the tough slog through treatment began. Surgery then chemotherapy.

Sue amazed us with her ability to work on her PhD while going through treatment. But though she did her best to put on a brave face, there were bleak moments. We tried to look for ways to bring a smile to her face. Shopping for shoes always worked. Planning for the baby also helped, and before you knew it, friends and family were rejoicing at her baby shower. With truly dramatic timing, Sue went into labour at the shower and left the party early.

We were elated the day Elona was born. Because she was premature there was some caution attached to the joy, but soon it was declared, "All is well". We celebrated her arrival. A nurse in Elona's unit joked that both mum and baby were bald. Being the protective aunt and sister I responded with the words, "It wasn't my sister's choice to be bald". Over the next many months we enjoyed babysitting Elona, which enabled Sue to rest or spend time with Kristof.

Summer came and another visit to my family doctor in early July reaffirmed my good health. It was a stunning blow when, less than two months later, Dr Callaghan looked me in the eye and told me I had breast cancer. I looked straight at him and said, "Okay, let's talk about a game plan". He was a bit surprised at my business-like approach to the diagnosis, but I had just spent the last 10 months supporting my sister so I knew what was coming my way.

While I was going through chemotherapy I asked again for genetic testing. This time they had enough evidence to support my request. I wasn't completely shocked when I received the news I tested positive for the BRCA II gene too. Sue and I both needed to know the truth, as did other members of our immediate and extended family. Cousins in Winnipeg all tested negative. My uncle was positive, as was, it turned out, my late father, because my mother was negative for the gene. Obviously, more testing lies ahead for our family in the future.

Cancer has impacted us. It has affected our family in so many ways. But cancer does not define us. We have the hearts of champions, and we see ourselves as champions as we band together to fight the fight.

Sandra Huculak
Sue Lawrence's sister
October 2015

PREFACE

This is my raw, unpolished, cancer story.

In the following pages you will find my unedited journal entries from the few weeks prior to being diagnosed with breast cancer until October 2015. I chose to publish my writing this way so you can hear my voice as it was then, during the days of torment, when I was in my most vulnerable state. Today, I am in a very different position, distant and safe from turmoil – healthy and happy. My reconstructed breasts are museum pieces. They have no feeling, only form, and they hang like plastic lemons on my chest wall. My old breasts were small and filled with shame. But my nipples were marvelous. And I miss them.

In June 2015, I arranged to see Alma Boerland, holder of a needle of dreams. She tattooed me a glorious pair of new nipples. They look splendid! They are like a painting on my chest – a painting which gives me deep pleasure. I have a carnal conduit now.

My dream is for this book to be a flare shot high into the sky signalling for all cancer patients and their families to feel whatever they want to feel with their cancer. It's yours. Writing this book has given me peace and freedom. May it bring the same to you.

Sue Lawrence
Delft, Netherlands
March 2016
www.suelawrence.co

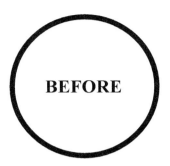

BEFORE

In October 2001, I moved to London, England from Canada to work at a university on a globalization and health project – the project was my ticket to understanding the world. I didn't. Instead, I had a good time being single in a big city. Before moving to London I had been married, divorced and lived a sheltered life as a nurse. I had no idea there were more than two types of cheese in the world (orange for cheddar and white for mozzarella). Cheese was just the beginning of my discoveries. I shared a four-story, worn-down flat in North London with three worldly-wise women who loved to celebrate and throw parties.

I met Kristof, a sweet Belgian, at one of our parties. His snails turned my head. We threw a French themed party. Everyone brought baguettes and Brie. Kristof brought snails in butter presented in little white pots.

He left the party early and forgot his pots. For the next year, he pursued my roommate to get his pots back. She had left the country. When his pots were finally returned to him via me, he began asking me for coffee and to eat fruit on the rooftop of the school. I took this to mean he was interested in me. He wasn't. He was just being friendly. It was at another party, six months later, that I suggested we dance. Kiss. He went along with it in his jovial way. It wasn't until a few days later he realized he liked me. That was in February 2005.

We moved in together in the fall of 2005. Our love nest was the bottom flat in Finsbury Park on the same road where my mother grew up. It came with a concave, squeaky bed, a table, three chairs, and Italian neighbours who shared their home-made sausage with us. My PhD started in January 2007.

I was at the beginning of a study to understand mental health risk and resilience factors in Israeli youth. In a pragmatic decision, we decided we preferred to stay together than be apart. He proposed in February 2007 during dinner at the restaurant in the British Museum, under its immense domed roof. My fingers were cold as they opened the red polka dotted boxes, each one smaller than the last. The final red sack held a pound store ring. We arrived in Israel in June 2007 and organized our wedding from the dark, cockroach-infested room we rented in Tel Aviv. We were getting married in Edmonton, Canada where all my family lived.

Kristof was finishing his PhD in Water and Sanitation when we married. He landed a job with International Resource Centre (IRC) shortly thereafter. A talented scientist with a passion for complexity, Kristof is often traveling to places needing water – Bangladesh, Burkina Faso, Mozambique.

Kristof was 42 when he proposed. He said he wanted children. At 35, I figured it would take me a year or so to become pregnant so I came off the pill. Elona was conceived in the heat of that Tel Aviv summer. She was a surprise and, in retrospect, a gift. Married on September 1, we headed out on a kayaking trip in British Columbia. There, on our floating chalet, we found a lump in my breast.

I have made additions to the journal entries only to make it clearer for you, dear reader. The journal entries are unedited. *Italics* indicate additional information to make the text clearer.

DURING

23 September 2007

Newly married and prior to diagnosis. We did not have a permanent home and neither of us had permanent jobs. We lived with my mother in Edmonton while we organized the wedding. We stayed with her during cancer treatment for financial reasons and emotional support.

There's a slight pressure when you start a new page. Daunting knowing that you should fill this first, fresh sheet with solid thoughts of inspiring, riveting text. So I am starting on the second page and reassuring myself that this diary is for my thoughts and no one judges them but me.

So this is the situation... I'm two months or so pregnant, queasy, dizzy and trying to concentrate on PhD stuff. Our future, my, our, newly married future is more unsure than it's ever been. Or perhaps the added responsibility of being a parent changes the weight of decisions. Childcare is my concern. Who will take care of the baby while I work? Can I count on Kristof? To an extent yes. But I imagine I'll need at least four hours of solid work time a day to get things done. How? It's a strange predicament to be homeless and jobless in this big world. Knowing we have a globe beneath our feet cushions some of my worries. Knowing I'm surrounded by women, families who have stepped here before me, is reassuring. It will work out somehow. It's nice to be married to Kristof. It's not a change or sense of security as before. I know that I've committed to him for life and I, we, need, must, should, treat each other well or it eats at intimacy. It's been a generous time. Friends have given and given and given and I feel spoiled with love and support. Wendy and John – days of thinking and rest and worry. Feeling safe enough to cry my eyes out. What a honeymoon! Days with Tena eating and laughing and just being blessed with so many great friends.

The wedding itself was perfect for us. Cosy, casual, laid back, fun, filled with people we love and who love us. *Yofi!* (Hebrew for great.)

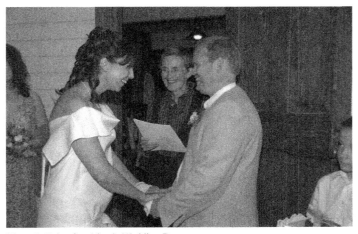

Photo 1: Kristof and Sue's Wedding Day

2 October 2007

After we found the lump on our honeymoon, Kristof pushed me to see a doctor before we returned to Tel Aviv. I thought it was just hormones. I didn't have an inkling of what was happening when the family doctor urgently made an appointment for an ultra-sound. Nor did I give it a second thought when the ultrasound technicians whispered to each other and then made an urgent appointment for a breast biopsy that afternoon. At the breast clinic, I recall a dark blue examination table and a big white machine with Philips™ on it as the doctor pricked a needle of tissue from my breast. Full of myself, I was babbling on to the doctor about going to Israel this week. She said,

"You'd better make other plans... you have an 80% chance of having breast cancer." I struggled to sit up to breathe. She showed me what was in the needle. It was a thin white worm of tissue. Kristof and I sat in a dark grey room with lighted panels for looking at x-rays while the doctor explained what was going to happen next. I was to see a surgeon to confirm diagnosis and to plan treatment options. My head stayed in that dark grey room for days.

I might have breast cancer. It's absurd and scary and unreal and very real. Grounded and flying away at the same time. It was a crazy day of doctors and nurses who went out of their way to help me out. I am grateful for all this help. But now I'm alone with my small, helpless breasts with which I had never really been at peace. And now they grow womanly and swollen with hormones and ironically rebel from their former bitter owner. I am alone with me. I'm picturing what will happen next. Will I go under anesthesia? Radiation? Chemotherapy?

How is my body building a baby and battling cancer at the same time? I will feed and water me and take extra good care of me. There's much work to be done. Fear, worry, sadness, loss, bewilderment. This morning, before the diagnosis, I was only pregnant.

I am surprised by it. Never thought I'd be at risk. I wonder which risk factor set me over the edge? I'm curious. Or what environmental hazard I ingested or was exposed to that triggered it. I wonder if I'll have a cancer that I can survive from. I don't want to die yet. Especially not leaving Kristof alone to raise our son/ daughter. My head swims with just about everything it can cram into itself. I want to feel something other than this pain. Tomorrow there will be more things to feel and think about. Tonight. I just have this tumour in my breast and all its baggage to keep me from sleeping.

What is keeping me awake? It's dark and silent and I'm alone. Do I start believing in God more? Do I start praying? It doesn't feel right. I hope everything will be okay. I hope I will be okay. I have hope.

3 October 2007

I've sunk into a sad darkness wanting to be free. This morning it occurred to me that this grief was mine and mine alone and that I could feel what I liked, when I liked. When I was grieving Dad, I felt restrained by society's restrictions. I was sad and wanted to wail and cry for days and be held. Instead, I bottled it up and hid away because none of my friends at the time knew how to deal with grief. So I kept it to myself.

And I did very stupid things in the process to feel something other than sadness. But this is all mine to cry and feel whatever I feel. Today it's still shock but more sadness and worry. Once I know what's happening, maybe then I can feel a bit better? Those I've told have been so supportive and I feel blessed.

4 October 2007

It's confirmed. I have breast cancer. Rationalising and reasoning myself out of it. It's not that bad. I feel profoundly sad and concerned about myself and the baby. This poor little soul is fighting for life and I'm fighting for mine too. This heavy weight is attached to my body, holding my heart down, holding my heart down.

Our surgeon was a young, hip guy who bounced into the room. He made a big fuss about Kristof's accent, his scruffiness and his international experience. He gave me the option of abortion, but we didn't take it. Because we have separate blood systems, Elona would not be exposed to chemotherapy. She was at risk of being born premature because the chemotherapy would stop hormones that sustain my pregnancy. Our oncologist was Dr Katia Tonkin, a straight talking, no bullshit Englishwoman. We had an amazing team of doctors who we saw almost every day. One day pregnancy, one day cancer. We were not going to start chemotherapy until Elona was 26 weeks. If I went into labour, she would survive.

8 October 2007

I'm overwhelmed with thoughts and emotions, worries and fear, anger sadness revulsion with my changing body, betrayed, lost. I'm in pain today and it disgusts me. I'm nauseated by it. My body is bloating from food and shrinking from disease. I run now to get away from the body. I prided myself on my strength and fitness fighting conformity to big-breasted thinness, happy and strong in myself and now I am covered in a thick film of fat and hormones that is aching and straining with disease. Will I have no breast? Will I be deformed? How will I cope with no hair for a few months? How will the baby be? How will he survive? Will he be okay? How do I get my body to survive?

I feel robbed of myself and who I am and what I do. On hold, my own life rests on someone else's words and plans, based on the changes within my small breast.

I was told, well-meaningly, that I shouldn't wear underwired bras as it restricts blood flow. And I see it in your eyes that you think I'm partially to blame for this tumour. It's me, my bras, those cigarettes and glasses of wine and having breasts in the first place that brought this on. I resent the last remark as I barely had them and I was they were just beginning to accept my body/ breasts for what they are, then this invasion alters and changes my perception of myself again. It's all about me.

What will they tell me? Will any of it be what I want to hear? The moment she said I had an 80% chance of having breast cancer, I lost hope of hearing happier news.

Anything he recommends, I will have to endure. Anything from a simple lumpectomy and treatment to mastectomy. I'll carry the wound, endure the treatment, have the story, lose the hair, vomit, worry about the baby.

The view changes from self-absorbed to wide angle. There are worse atrocities done to people and many women go through this. But it doesn't make me feel connected to them statistically, or better off, or thankful for receiving this suffering rather than another.

I'm barely listening to the rest of the world, mildly tuning in from time to time. I resent this cancer coming at a time like this. I've wanted so long to be pregnant, wanted a child, wanted to enjoy being pregnant, nurturing my growing child. I feel robbed of this joy, this tumour has muscled in on the natural progression of this little life. Taken my centre stage, the starring role given to the tumour rather than baby. I am a vessel for this baby, a receptacle for this tumour and a bloated soft shell, rounded and curved.

17 October 2007

Tomorrow I lose my entire left breast. After years of abuse and feeling bad about it, it's saying goodbye and I'm saying goodbye to it. It's sad, scary and makes me mad to lose it. All my hopes of being a mum and feeding my baby with my breast are gone. I may not be able to have another baby after this one. There is a chance I may not live through this cancer. But these answers won't be answered until after the pathology report.

The cancer doctor was good but she made it known that she knew best. And did. She was worried about my survival. Being worried about baby's survival was something she said I was wired to do. But this wiring was not always best for decision making.

I woke up angry, gritting my teeth and ready to attack. Angry at the world for being in this predicament. Angry for being robbed of a normal pregnancy.

And what of my PhD? Something I had been looking forward to doing and learning and revelling in – pushed aside for a while.

18 October 2007

Goodbye breast. After all these years you are full, rounded and beautiful with life. I love you and I'm sorry to see you go. I love you Sue, I love you Kristof and I love you baby.

I had grade 3 invasive ductal carcinoma of the left breast and had a complete mastectomy. If I had not been pregnant, I would have had a lumpectomy with chemotherapy and radiation.

20 October 2007

I have a big, long, ugly scar where my breast used to be. The size and ugliness of the scar equals the fear, the anger, and the sadness that was in it. Now that the cancer is 'gone' I feel better, like a weight is lifted. We've gotten over the first hurdle.

27 October 2007

I am breastless. Empty space. Disturbing, mutant. It's not my badge of honour. Victory. Though I don't mind sporting it to show others the reality of breast cancer. The past few days have been painful and I've worked hard to shit it out and be cheerful. Today, there's less pain and I'm tired. Tired of this ugly drain dangling from me, of doctors and decisions and waiting. I am, as usual, impatient to get on with life and work. I am tired of talking about cancer and pregnancy. Tired of it framing my daily existence. But I suppose it's better than last year – unemployed, poor and living off food from the Pound Shop (Dollar Store).

29 October 2007

Heavy with anger, sadness, betrayal. Heavy tears sit on my chest. It aches and aches. Pain here, pain there. The continual telling of the story is tiring and reminds me of what is ahead. I feel very alone in this. It's happening to me and those around me sympathise and support and offer what they can. I am alone, bewildered and tired.

I've stopped talking to Kristof, a childish thing. But all I hear from him are counterarguments and pedantic details and corrections and no support just a battling wall that I want to stay away from right now. I don't have the strength to argue or defend myself or fight. All my strength is going into… ? What? Baby? Staying fed, watered, healthy, keeping sane and calm. Seeking out people who make me feel good and staying away from those who make me feel bad.

3 November 2007

I am making a choice. Preserving my life or my child's. Flooding my body with chemicals goes against my instinct to protect my child. Kristof asked me to take care of his baby... I am flooding it with chemicals to keep myself alive. I am guilty and selfish. The boundary between my child and I are drawn. Do other mothers make this distinction so soon? As we grow an unborn life form within our bellies do we automatically connect with this being? This being that we must love and protect by the very nature and instinct of our being. Do we, through self-preservation, make this separation at some point? My child. Me. The I in my child is me.

I have given my breast, my dignity, my health to cancer. The rest of my body is nurturing the child. My head sits atop it all and watches, questions, grieves the loss of this and that and tries to bridge the body, the baby, the breast and the lost soul.

In a few short weeks our lives were devastated, shattered, fell apart, the path twisted and went off in a direction unfathomable. How did we get here?

How did we get to this place? And then another type of guilt comes in. Which wrong turn did I take? The 'what' and 'how' and 'how much' and 'how often' or 'not enough' did I do or not do to have this change of direction of wills occur? Was it the red wine? The occasional cigarette? The not having babies early enough? I exercised, ate red meat, stayed up late, worried. I lived fiercely, recklessly and something in that equation came to this. The 'what I am' and 'what I did' or didn't do turned a cell bad. Its mutation setting off a chain reaction for others to follow. They gained speed and force and went wild and big. Became ambitious and wanted to see new paths of my body. Thankfully we managed to get there in time to stop the journey from ending badly.

I watch baby grow from my changing, lopsided body. The glowing, life-giving body of pregnancy I admired in friends is, in me, marked by a gash across my chest of an adolescent span of skin.

But Mummy has to live, to protect her child, to guide it, nurture it and be its guide. I won't give up this task. Self-preservation for me and for my child. The I in my child is me.

8 November 2007

I tell them I'm fine. It's what they want to hear. In their minds this is over now that the tumour is gone. It's so not over.

Focus on surviving, getting through. I have no doubt I'll survive. It's the process that's killing me. It's isolating and lonely and I feel like I have to defend myself at any moment. The *Get Well Soon* – I have cancer. When's *Soon*?

Cancer shapes my world. There are so many of us with breast cancer. I hope to find a friend in this growing pile of victims. I don't feel sick yet I can't do the things I love to do… run. This isn't my life.

10 November 2007

I didn't realize how proud I am until now. This experience feels like an invasion of my dignity, a personal insult. My dignity, sense of self, altered, invaded, ripped apart. A grave injustice to myself. Bury myself in that grave. My breast taken away casually, quickly, with a quick nod to the doctor of its importance, leaving me raw, exposed, grieving. I was flat chested before but this is extreme.

Gerry's offhand comment on in his opinion all women

who cook on television touched a raw nerve, well many of them. The breast's importance roars in my ears and eyes. I didn't measure up before and I certainly don't now. I have no strength to be defiant.

Gerry is my brother in law. He is a lovely guy and it really was just an offhand comment.

17 November 2007

On a recent quick trip through London, UK, I was bombarded by the numerous images of cleavage hanging around billboards, street corners, coffee shops and every magazine on the shelf. Can I have cleavage with only one breast? Would the bra engineers design a sexy, or pretty mastectomy bra, please?

Mastectomy bras are sold in chemist shops not lingerie shops. Lingerie stores dangle pretty bras adorned with lace, silk, and satin. Enticing you to seduce someone with your assets. Mastectomy bras resemble slingshots in white or beige polyester, cotton blends to bring out the grandmother in you. If this ugly trend has something to do with the fact that most woman who get breast cancer are in their late 40s, 50s and 60s, and therefore may not always opt to buy sexy lingerie, then I'm outraged they have given up their sexy lingerie. When does this happen? Mind you, I can see the lack of enthusiasm in playing the 'get your attention' game especially when your priorities are split between a myriad other more important things.

When I wear my polyester/ cotton-blend weapon, complete with my beanbag boob, I feel like I'm wearing a bulletproof vest, arming me for battle. There is a sense of Amazonian woman in this, this one-sided warrior, face the world smiling while you mourn the loss of things you held so dear – breasts, babies, and youth.

Shopping for a prosthesis is another experience in itself. How about a slab of rubber to carry around in your ugly bra, so you can look 'normal'? From what other women have said, they're hot, and heavy. I have chosen to use a beanbag to simulate my boob. It feels alien so I find myself poking it in public if a bean is out of place. So even though it 'looks' real, it's not to me. To be honest, most days I can't be bothered looking real. I don't fit into this breast-obsessed society. Don't get me wrong, not donning the boob is not some perverse attempt to get attention, or be a walking bill-board for breast cancer awareness. Looking down, it's a shallow place, my heart is closer to the world, not stronger, not dignified, just pulsing under my skin. Weary, the Amazonian image doesn't fit me either.

I will be going for reconstruction surgery next year, a process that will take six months, as they have to fill my flat chest first to stretch the skin and make space for an implant. Then it will be six weeks of post-surgery recovery. All of this to look normal, to sport two bouncing globes of flesh, one mine, one the health care system's. Afterwards, I'll be able to wear any bra I like or no bra for that matter. I'll be able to squish them up and together and hell, anywhere I please with today's lingerie technology. I wonder whether I'll care by that time.

I apologize if this section is not in the correct order. I didn't edit any of the diary entries. They came straight from the written page. Shopping for a prosthesis bra and beanbag occurred a few weeks after the first mastectomy. I still have that beanbag boob if anyone needs it.

November 2007

Kristof and I went to Israel, Belgium and then the UK to organize things for my PhD and to tell Kristof's parents the news. I made these entries sometime in this trip. We met up with a lot of friends and family during this time.

me this will make me stronger. How do ? Is there some sort of before and after test ına do to see what's stronger? Like what? My endurance for pain and suffering? My ability to handle stress? My hatred of myself? I can tell you one thing that's going to be stronger is my dislike for people like you.

18 November 2007

What will I need all this strength for? What do I do with it? What does a stronger person do differently than one who is not strong? How do you measure it? I won't be able to have any more babies and I will go into menopause. I miss my breast. I hate my prosthesis bra and my prosthesis. I'm scared of chemo. I'm scared of Tamoxifen. I am cold with it all.

How do I hold my head up and get out of bed? I don't want to face the world. But I do. Every day. There's a big lump in my chest of something I'm holding in. It's a scream? It is an ear-piercing, blood curdling scream of insanity. I can't take any more of this. I can't handle anything more than this. Stop please.

Even though I'm happy I'm going away, I carry all these emotions with me. I can't escape from them. I can't hide, push them away/ down, and ignore them.

It's my life, the one I'm trying to live. The one-line emails from friends of how worried they are. I can't sum up in one line all that this entails. I feel like a big human, a larger than life one right now. Messy. The ball in my chest is rising. It's not a scream. It's panic. What do I do with all this? I'm going crazy with this swirling mass of stuff. It's tangled and painful and overwhelming. How do I do this? I'm so angry too. The ball in my chest is weariness. I'm tired of holding my head up, moving forward, living. That ball in my chest is everything, all at once.

We went to Israel to wrap up things for the PhD, and Belgium to see Kristof's parents.

22 November 2007

(Sixth anniversary of Dad's death)

I was thinking about you this morning. Thinking about loss and aches and how when you lose something of yourself or someone, nothing fills the ache left behind. Not tears or anger or rage or sadness or a thousand prayers. It's just an ache that stays. I find that people don't want to see my suffering. They're uncomfortable with it. They'd rather see me happy and strong and reward me with praise when I perform. I am a crazy, sad seal. Suffering and sadness are hard to look at, harder to take in.

I want so much to be held by something bigger and larger than this ache that consumes me. Is it God I'm calling? It is God I'm calling. Something that is comfortable with this ugliness of me, that no wants to see. I don't understand this idea of not wanting to see this side of people. It's reality and it's all around us. Why is my pain so hard for them to bear? I spend energy making sure they see the happy, strong side of me because that's what they want to see and it's easier. I understand social niceties and that there is a time and a place for pain... but where is it? Is there a room we can go where we can let it all hang, fall away and let us just be? It's not that ugly, it's just pain, sorrow, sadness. Nothing new, sometimes overwhelming.

You, me, the ones who suffer are wondering around with gaping holes of ick. We nod politely to each other and smile knowingly. Maybe there is a room we can go to for people who've been there and back and we know that sometimes we don't show this sadness to the world. It's a private matter, not for show. I had some pictures taken of my belly and my scar. I wonder what propelled me to do this? A grotesque display of rage, suffering, humiliation and anger. No one sees my tears or wants to see them, so I show them defiantly with my scar. Humans are fascinated by horrors and it's easier than seeing suffering, but it doesn't satisfy me, it just leaves me as empty and sad as before. There is no comfort. I know I wanted to mark this time in my life in a picture. This time of my life won't be forgotten and I want to honour it by being recorded. My gift to myself and my pain, my acknowledgment that I know this is hard.

Hope rests in this baby and yet, I don't want the weight of life on her shoulders just yet. It's my job to protect her from the bad things in life. And it started sooner than most mothers have to do mothering. So she is an aside… the work of my future… and the work of now is to keep Kleenex companies in business.

We found out we were having a girl during one of the routine ultrasound appointments.

20 December 2007

The travelling cancer show is back. It was great to see everyone but I was far more interested in their lives. And I had to talk about mine. Talking about it so much when it feels so huge and overwhelming. I don't know who I am supposed to be.

I'm scared, sad and tired. I don't want cancer. I don't want to do this. I am emotional. How do I do this? Does being pregnant make this more huge? Am I supposed to take losing my breast to cancer lightly? Stoically?

I don't want to hear advice or people telling me anything. My nerves are raw and on edge. I imagine God or someone strong and powerful cradling me in their hands, gently, lovingly, nurturing me. Let me curl up and cry and sleep and just be comforted. Mother me.

I had my first chemotherapy on December 24, I was 26 weeks pregnant. I was due to have six chemo sessions, about three weeks apart.

8 January 2008

Will this marriage last? Now is not the best time to think about it but I don't feel any connection or closeness. He does his work, his face stuck in a computer. There's no nurturing or compassion, just distance. I asked for reassurance, long ago, but I didn't get this either. This is too much for this fledgling relationship. Living with my mother, overwhelmed with change. My body altered. Sadness. Him not getting it. Him being selfish?

Why do I have to do the emotional work? My husband rejects me, is repulsed by me, or is indifferent, or is busy and selfish? Will I have to find the strength to leave him too? Prepare myself financially first? Do I feel emotionally abandoned by him in a time of need so I shut myself off and pull away to protect and save myself first?

I was so in love with him and he pulled away and now I pull away. I can remain friends, it's what I do better with men anyway. I can be respectful for the sake of our child. This is me being stubborn. I resent that. Like it's my fault he pulled away. I can do the loving for both of us, it's not my job. Right now, I have to take care of me and baby and that's all. So put that into action and let go of anger, hurt, anxiety, whatever else is keeping you up at night, robbing you of energy and rest. You know you. Boy, I wish I had two breasts. Be gentle with yourself. Be so very gentle with me. I want to be somewhere beautiful, peaceful, somewhere where I'm loved, around people who will warmly, open heartedly love me, embrace me, hold me, cuddle me, help me hold my soul together. Help me to nurture my ragged soul.

9 January 2008

My hair fell out this morning. Vulnerable, ugly, sad, drained, weary. Why am I doing this to the baby? Is it really necessary? If I hear one more story of someone who survived breast cancer and is fine now, I will punch them in the nose. I feel like I've betrayed my baby already. Guilt. Putting my life in front of hers.

17 January 2008

The second phase of chemo felt like the worst hangover. Today my bowels feel like they're falling out of my ass. But it feels good to have a shower.

My sister said how I have the cutest head and I'm doing fine.

Kristof and I attended our first prenatal class on February 22. My vision of my birth was for it to be natural and relaxing, perhaps sip a small beer like they do in the UK. Where I got this idea, I don't know. I even went so far as to ask the nurse at the prenatal class if I could have a beer during labour. Her face twisted and there was a long pause. She said the doctor could prescribe alcohol if necessary. I found this to be an odd answer. Prescribe alcohol? Only much later did I realize she thought I was an alcoholic and needed to have it. During the class, my back started to hurt. And this backache continued off and on over Saturday and Sunday. My waters broke on Sunday at 9.30 pm. Kristof timed my contractions as he drove over icy Canadian streets. We didn't speak about how close together they were. I arrived at the hospital fully dilated. Elona was born Sunday February 24, 2008 at 11.05 pm. Because I had gone into menopause with chemotherapy, she was six weeks premature. She spent around three weeks in the neo-natal intensive care unit where she learned to breathe and eat.

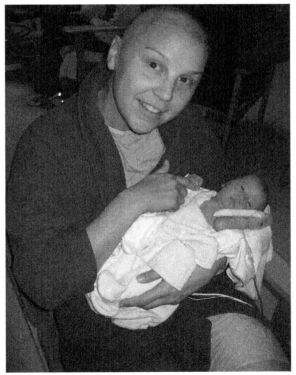

Photo 2: Iona and I in the Misericordia Hospital, Edmonton, Canada. Elona is a few days old.

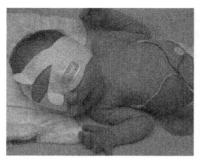

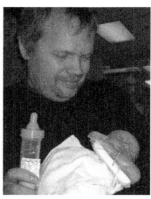

Photo 3 (above): Elona under the blue light
– a few hours old.
Photo 4 (right): Kristof, the proud papa.

February 2008

Can you have a honeymoon in your mother-in-law's house?

No. We stayed at my mother's place prior to the wedding. Once we were diagnosed, we moved in. We lived in my mother's house for my treatment. For financial reasons, we had no other choice. My mother was a tremendous help to me especially when Elona was born. She happily took over feeding and holding while I slept.

My husband, already feeling stripped of an ability to feel effective, was rendered even more useless by his mother-in-law. We learned we could survive anything if you decide not to feel. My husband shut himself in the basement with his computer. He emerged when it was dinner time. Talking to each other is NOT a solution if either of you are on cell-destroying drugs. Leave the deep and meaningfuls until at least two years after treatment when your brain cells are back and/ or you live in your own space.

5 March 2008

Dear Elona,

I wanted to have you a decade before I had you. I dreamed about being a mother. And with my only chance, I flooded you with chemicals. You were foremost in my mind and the oncologist warned me that if I didn't take care of me, you might not have a mother. Losing a breast – well, it's a mighty loss, especially as I wanted to breastfeed you. That was taken away. Here you are, ten days old, struggling to eat and breathe. Today, I watched the nurse bring you back from one of your apnea episodes. You went white and limp and the nurse rubbed your back until you came alive again. I love you so much this minute and it pains me to my soul to hear you cry, watch you struggle. I would give you my life if you needed it. Now there is no oncologist telling me to live to raise you. Now I only want to live and be strong and grow so I can raise you. Today I want to live for you, you sweet strong little life.

28 March 2008

In the dark. There's a lot of self-pity and sadness with this. I hate the pitying looks people give me when I wear that skull cap. I'm tense, in pain, don't feel like myself. My arm hurts, my ass hurts. I'm dry and ugly. It's an effort keeping this together. Maybe I should just fall apart for a few days. Relax and be in pain. I want to go and hide in a hole for a while. Be away from everyone and mirrors. The baldness is no longer unique. I just have cancer. I spend a lot of energy trying to keep going, to keep my head high despite vulnerability. I feel very alone in this. I don't feel listened to or nurtured. Nurture me, make a fuss. It's what I need.

When you have cancer, people tell you about their sad stories. Do they think it makes me feel better to hear of worse cancer? Am I competing here? Is one's suffering weighted differently? Who gets more pity? Well, I don't want pity. I want to be nurtured and no one has presented that. No one's offered that save for a few, very few.

9 April 2008

The last days of 36.

When I embarked on this year, I was playful, light in

mind and body and feeling gorgeous, fit and fiery. Little did I know I was carrying a Stage III cancer in my left breast and most of the year would be spent surviving it. It's been hell, but what I'm finding in these last days of being 36 is that, once again, in my grief, I can't speak about it. Tearful with the oncologist, I was told I was emotional because of the chemotherapy. NO! I'm emotional because I have a cancer that has a high chance of recurring. And because I was pregnant with cancer and had to give my first, dear, child chemotherapy. And had to parade bald and ugly to the world with my head held high in an attempt to survive. And had to fight to still be me despite all the threats to myself.

I bought a book on how to deal with cancer afterwards and so many of the words ring true. I've lost friends and can't speak to some friends because they just don't get it. I carry something different inside me now. I do feel like a survivor, but I'm in the process of surviving now. There's a 20 percent chance of it coming back and that is where the hope rests. I learned a lot about hope this year. I hadn't really felt hope until it was all I had to fall back on. I hoped I wouldn't die, I hoped my much longed for baby would be allowed to stay. I hoped the chemotherapy wouldn't hurt her. I hoped the chemotherapy wouldn't hurt me. I hoped I would survive. I hoped the surgery wouldn't hurt her, I hoped I would survive the surgery. I hoped Kristof would still love me even though I was no longer whole, but a diseased, bald, Amazonian who can't shoot an arrow to save her life. I hope still.

I suppose you don't need hope when everything's going well and you're trucking along buying groceries and doing chores and working and stressing about your stresses. Having to live hoping, with every piece of yourself, with your soul aching on hope, is really tiring. My soul seems to exercise a little bit on it every day. That tiny bit of myself that thinks of cancer every day and with those thoughts, I hope I don't have to think about cancer every day again. Here's hoping.

In the last days of 36, I feel deeper in myself than I've ever been and more grateful for life and our life than ever before. I have my life, my daughter's, my husband's life. In the last days of 36, I'm preparing for another round of chemotherapy, knowing how shitty it makes me feel, reconciling that it's for the best and dreading it all the same. I am dreading it and it's a shitty birthday present in one sense and it's the best birthday present to myself. Give me the life preserving drugs that make me feel like I want to die.

12 April 2008

New pieces of me. I looked in the mirror the other day and saw a plucked chicken – pale, sickly, prickly. My soul is grasping for a way to me. Or is lost or in pain, bewildered, forlorn, in need of compassion, nurturing, love. I am not who I was before.

Ravaged soul, ravaged body. I had cancer, chemotherapy, mastectomy, a baby, a pregnancy and a marriage. The pieces are all there and they are new pieces of my life.

Spoke with miracle Marianne – mother miracle Marianne. She gently told me that I don't have to subject myself to walking around bald every day. It's true – it's only for days when I'm feeling strong. I don't have to be strong and brave every day.

I met miracle Marianne in the recovery room after my last chemotherapy. We have been close friends ever since. She has had breast cancer twice and receives Herceptin to keep a tumour that's tucked in her chest at bay.

In June 2008, we moved back to Belgium as Kristof started a job in the Netherlands and he had an apartment we could live in, in Belgium. We stayed in Belgium until September 2008 when we moved to

Israel so I could finish my data collection for my PhD. My mother joined us in Israel to help take care of Elona while Kristof and I worked. We left Israel February 2009, went to Belgium for a few months and then returned to Canada in June 2009 for breast reconstruction.

Breast reconstruction entailed inserting a balloon into my chest wall, which would, over a period of weeks, be filled with water in order to stretch the skin.

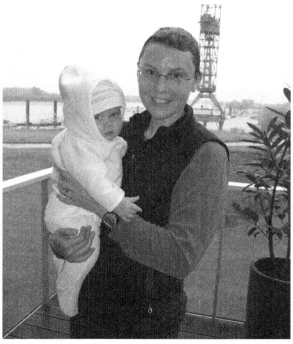

Photo 5: Elona and I after my first run (Elona is six months old).

My sister Sandra was diagnosed with breast cancer in September 2008, while we were in Israel and unable to support her. She underwent a double mastectomy and breast reconstruction over the course of a year and a half. She underwent genetic testing and found that she had the breast cancer gene. She also had her ovaries and fallopian tubes removed as preventative measures.

I tested positive too, and decided to have my right breast removed. Kristof, Elona and I stayed in Canada from June 2009 to June 2010 in order to do all the reconstruction surgeries. I decided not to have my ovaries out at this time as we were still considering having more children. Once again, we stayed with my mother in her house.

8 April 2009

The last days of 37.

I am reluctant to start this entry this year. It's because the year was heavy and long-stretched over rocks, my skin, it was that painful. I had chemotherapy days before my birthday and was in a fog for a week. The fog lifted, briefly, my eyes pained from the sun, dripping with mucus, hairless, limp, a baby bird without the grace of new life. My last chemo was April 29, and Marianne was there to celebrate with me. Chemo-therapy smells of rubber bands and it still sticks at the back of my nose. I want to retch. As they pulled the needle out I felt as much triumph as I could muster amidst my feeling sorry for myself. There wasn't a lot to be proud of. It was all a terrible struggle to keep my head together, as everything fell apart.

I didn't want to leave Edmonton and the safety of friends and family. Alone, back in Temse, Kristof away, Mimi (my mother-in-law) not understanding, I was left to grieve my losses alone. I felt abandoned, dejected, misunderstood and terribly sad. The summer was succulent and warm, breathing life into me – the hairless baby bird who was angry at her plight. Elona and I went for daily walks to Teilrode, 45 minutes of listening to birds, watching spring evolve.

It took a while to calm down, to settle into myself, to not feel like a mutant. No one considered me a mutant – but I felt alien to myself – what had just happened to me was still open and raw. The chemicals were still in me, I could feel them, feel my body betraying me. Going out into the world, I felt exposed and vulnerable – like everybody suspected something was odd about me –because I felt odd about myself. I was not yet me.

Looking back, I see it was adjusting to, well, a life with cancer, and motherhood. Two mutually exclusive painful processes combined – a spin through a grinder, crushing everything so it no longer resembled itself.

I write a letter to myself at the eve of every birthday. This year we had moved from Canada to Belgium straight after chemotherapy and I began working on my PhD again. Temse and Teilrode are small towns in Belgium. Our apartment is in Temse.

15 February 2010

Seeing Elona so gentle and kind hooked up to heart monitors because of me and the drugs that kept me alive. I wouldn't be here without those drugs and she wouldn't be here without me. She makes me want to live. I am alive for her and she is alive from me.

Chemotherapy can affect the heart development of children exposed during utero. Elona is monitored every ten years for changes.

I had my right breast removed in March 2010. This surgery was also the first phase of breast reconstruction where they inserted an empty prosthesis under my chest wall, which they would slowly fill with saline.

30 March 2010

The last days of my right breast. For many reasons the left breast never had a send off. This time, I'd like to honor its presence and passing with some focused thoughts.

I never really liked the size and shape of my breasts and felt shame and embarrassment whenever I had to undress in front of others. What I loved, enjoyed, cherished about them and will miss dearly is the sensation in my nipples. Kristof treated them so well, his tongue makes them tingle and I will miss, miss, miss, miss this sensation so much. The surgery is six days away and I'm scared of what exactly. First, it was dying, which is still present. I'm glad I'm getting this mastectomy – it will be one less source of cancer to worry about. I will be happy – finally – with the size and shape of my breasts. But they're only for show. Their source of ecstasy will be gone. One of the things that feels good in life will be gone. In living, what makes us feel good becomes concentrated into few things.

The surgery brings back all the horrible memories of before. Chemo – viewing life through a straw of pain, sorry, grief. Do I need help with this? I find the cancer story slips out a lot – like I'm an oozing, emotional slut wanting to share my pain with everyone. I don't like this at all. The pain needs a proper out. An outlet, a place to honor it so that I don't continue to spill my guts at strange, inappropriate moments like the Dior counter lady. A shrine to pain? A box of horrors? A container of cancer chaos?

This started out as an ode to my breast – but I don't know what else to say to it, to me, who is holding it, who is feeling bad for all the bad feelings I've had for so long.

I want to give my nipple a royal send-off but I'm not sure what that would entail – lots and lots and lots of fondling. Wish I could capture the feeling in a small Plexiglas box. Wish I could encase it in pieces of chocolate, which I could eat at a later date. My little nipple so small, inconspicuous to everyone but me. A small source of pleasure for mornings. What will I wake up to now? I am trading this lovely, sweet, nipple for a future guaranteed not to have cancer. Not to have to go through chemotherapy, radiation, not to hear those words. I am trading pleasure for something that may not happen, never happen. I may be cancer free but the odds are against me. So goodbye nipple. Thank you for all the pleasure you have given me. I will miss you. I will miss you so very much.

31 March 2010

Post surgery.

Well, it's done. My breasts are much smaller but fuller than before. They will be compact, good looking little breasts.

8 April 2010

The last days of 38.

Do you get back what you lose in some way? Is what you put into something, its depth/ breadth equal to the pain of losing it? Two new breasts with no feeling = two non-pretty breasts with feeling + cancer.

It's not logical, doesn't fit equations – is not tidy and symmetrical. I am so happy with my new breasts and no fear of breast cancer. I miss, terribly, my nipples. I ache for that sensation again. Never again. It's just gone.

23 April 2010

Met with Dr Tonkin. It was a pleasure to see her. She gave me her email address and asked me to keep in touch. I felt honored, touched and relieved because I felt the same way – I wanted to keep in touch with her too. She made sense and logic from a crazy horrible time. She said it was a terrible time.

She said I have to stay on the Tamoxifen to stop other tumours from growing. Plus, I have to get my ovaries out. She also said I had to watch out for osteoporosis, high blood pressure and high cholesterol because I'll be in menopause that much sooner than everyone else.

Sobering. I felt the edges of my life. Sharply defined and not some shifting blob of endless time. There will be an end to me and only a few will remember me.

15 June 2010

Elona tried to breastfeed from me. I was cradling her in my arms and she looked up at me and I knew what she wanted. She wanted to suckle. She pulled down my top and sucked from each breast. Strange that she knows this, she seems disappointed. Does she know she missed out? She must. She notices my Band Aids. It will be loss, a loss we'll share. Me for not being able to give, her for not being able to receive.

I don't feel afraid of death – no, that's a lie. I don't want to die just yet. I want to raise Elona. The more I get to know her, the more I am amazed at how strong and confident and outgoing she is. She is alive!

Vibrant! She shines. She has something within her that is strong, self-assured, clever and sensitive. If I die sooner than I'd like to, I believe she will shine out of loss. I believe she is strong in her soul and mind and will withstand not having me around.

Elona was two-and-a-half years old – healthy, happy, and always singing. The plastic surgeon who reconstructed my breast, the master breast maker Dr Campbell, said I should continue to wear surgical tape across my scars to reduce stretching. Elona saw these as 'owies'.

15 February 2012

For as long as I've been able I've wanted to give birth and breastfeed, wanted to give birth to the world my children, create my family. I had images of carrying children strapped to my hip, my breasts full of milk, other kids running around creating a noisy mess and me happy in the chaos and fun. It was going to be a fun life, lived close to the earth, close to my heart. The intervening years of divorce, moving to UK, took me away from those roots until I met Kristof. A few months after being engaged to Kristof, I went off the pill thinking it would take six months or more to get pregnant. About a month and a half after sending off wedding invitations, I was pregnant. I was smug in my fertileness. My body, my soul was ready and waiting to build this baby. When I was diagnosed with breast cancer at the end of the first trimester, and told I would have to have a mastectomy, I held onto the fact I had one breast left to nurture my child.

Chemotherapy started when I was in the second trimester. I gave birth to her after the second treatment and right before the third treatment (it was almost as if she knew she should come that weekend rather than wait until I was exhausted from chemo and could not push her out). She was six weeks premature and they whisked her away seconds after I saw her screaming, red, wet face. I wanted so much to hold her, to have her right next to me, to love her and it was such an ache, a terrible, terrible pain to have to stand on the other side of glass and watch her breathe, bathed in blue light. My right breast had filled up with milk. Could they sense how much hope and fulfillment was behind that question? Could I breastfeed? There were too many cancer-killing chemicals in my body for the breast milk to do any good.

It was deeply ironic that I, who longed to be an earth mother, had been bald, pumped up with chemicals, with only one breast, standing over the glass case that held my one and only child.

On Monday, I hand over my fallopian tubes with the full knowledge that this is the absolute end of any hope of the earth mother returning. I give fallopian tubes that may contain ovarian cancer to the gynecologists who will toss them casually into a container for hazard waste disposal. I tell you this – those gentle tubes are NOT a hazard and the only hazard they contain are my screams of a different dream for myself.

I was going to do a symbolic salute to my tubes, like I did my breast. In my mind I had sent my cancerous breast over a 50-foot waterfall. I feel like a bonfire, a huge, raging fire that's hot with my rage and contained pain. But I am going to go and buy some flower bulbs and plant them in my garden. There is life in death as there is death in life.

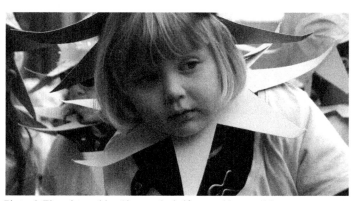

Photo 6: Elona is sunshine (three and a half years old years old)

7 September 2012

Having cancer is almost noble. As soon as you tell someone you have, or had, cancer – they think you're brave and courageous. A switch was not turned on when they told me I had cancer – a switch that suddenly filled me with strength and clarity and desire to live. I was dizzy with loss, lost in a hundred thoughts and worries, deep fear – I had never felt the end of my life before. It has an edge, and I am getting closer to it. Someday I will die. There was an inner force, but it was more to do with trying to keep from crying, screaming, laying in bed every day. It had nothing to do with being courageous. But because everyone tells you that you are brave, you hold yourself a little taller, you are a hero because you survived your own death. But then, all of us who are living should be heroes too. We're surviving death. Is the challenge then that whoever lives the longest, wins? Elderly people are trembling, fragile, they move through tumbling people with reluctance and they always look sad. Is it because our faces have fallen so far that they can't perk up into joy? I notice that about my own face, sinking into sorrow. When I don't feel sorrow, just living. The ideal would be to live a long, long time, healthy, sexy and firm – with no leaks or bent parts.

6 November 2012

Another month of all things pink gone by. It was at the back of my mind, but it didn't come fully forward. I love my breasts. I love their soft slope and heavy feel. I love the way my bra holds them, how the bra captures the curves. I always wanted breasts like this yet hid the desire from myself thinking I was way above this kind of conceit. Dammit! If I was honest, I wanted curves instead of the small breasts I had. I was so small that they didn't make pretty bras for me. And if they did, they came with a lot of padding, which rubbed in the idea that I didn't have enough. Was not enough. So I carried around that sense of inadequacy in a foam-filled cup.

I couldn't wait to have children so these breasts would grow, fill with fuel. My luscious, life giving curves! I was told in my leadership course to want things. I wanted larger breasts then. Perhaps it was tied to something deeper, a sense of loving myself. Three months into my first and only pregnancy, on our honeymoon floating in a cabin off the coast of Vancouver, the ice grey sea and the ice grey sky, reflecting ghoulishly shaped wood, I found that lump in my breast. Over a span of just three years, I had both breasts removed and reconstructed. I grin and say they are my booby prize for surviving.

24 February 2013

Five years ago tonight, Elona was born. She was born in my storm. She was born in bewilderment, being lost, resentful and stubborn. She was born. Elona Joy. There was even resentment over your name because Joy was from my own mother and we did not recognise the mother of your father. I can tell you I felt I had a right to name you 'joy' and connect you and me to my mother. You were hard born from my body, from my soul. My DNA locked with yours. Your soul entwined with mine from the beginning and forever more. And if you think that souls die and leave you – think again. They do not. I am still connected to my father. And you, Elona, will forever be connected to me. And I can say I am so very proud to be your mother. That all the criticism I think is felled upon me, falls away because I am so proud to have gotten through with you and me and our souls intact. And I hope to instil in you the passion I have for you, for living and being. I have lived so recklessly, sweetheart, so without mind-fulness. So without thinking. Just propelling myself forward in the direction my heart takes me. And maybe that is being soulful which is deeper than mindful so it's okay too. I got here, in this lovely house with your lovely father by not asking. By loving. And not knowing.

My dear, you are five today. You are so full of joy and wonderment. I want to capture you like a butterfly and hold all your beautiful moments still. To stand back and hold you to the light and be in amazement. You are a force. You are what a young woman should be. You are a child, full of precious time. Lived by painting, and playing and princess dresses and magic wands and fairy wings. My dear, you are five today. I so want it all to be okay for you. To be well. I hope to instil in you the strength and wisdom to live your life on your terms. That you must approve of you first. That all is okay. All is well dear, because all *is* well. The Universe holds me and you and all of us amongst fragile quivering threads of energy and we try and try and try to live. Live my love. Live. Live and be content as much as you can. All is well. It has taken me 42 years to learn this so don't be so hard on yourself if it takes you a while too. Please be kind to yourself and be kind to others as you would be kind to yourself.

Five years ago tonight you were born to me to take care of. I know in my deepest heart that I did not know how to do this, I did not know how to step into being your mother. That I was reluctant to be your mother – part of me was going through the motions, part of me was wanting to run out the door from fear. Fear of? It was a deep uncertainty. I was resentful at the world for giving you to me not the way I had planned, but with a bitter gift that was foremost in my mind. My life, my body. Consumed with myself, I could not get past myself to you. I wish I could have ripped open the blue glowing box that held your tiny, wired body and hold you to me like I wanted to so much. Deep in my heart, I wanted to love you so passionately from the first moment I saw you. And I had to let others decide how my interactions with you were going to be.

I so wanted to be alone with you. Alone with you and your wonderment and cry like every other mother does. Rich with hormones I wanted to bond. And I couldn't. I was standing in the way between you and me. It took me a long time to get rid of that anger and get to you. You, who had been there all the while, waiting patiently for me. Waiting for your mother to step into herself. My, you must have learned patience from an early age. We are all fragile souls so forgive me. Forgive me for all that I have warped you with, and turned you into, and not given you. Forgive me. I am learning too. And as you know now, I failed at the first lesson. Thank God your father was there and fell in love with you and took care of you right away. Your father is wonderful. Don't ever forget that. For all the things he isn't, he is so much more.

And I am the passionate artist soul that is flaky and flits and whines because I'm sensitive. And I have to be sensitive to touch all the parts of me that are hidden and I understand how things work because I have to pay attention to the small things inside me.

Five years ago tonight your little body embodied hope and wanting from a long time. Your 2500 grams of life held years of longing. What you are to me are stars and heaven and soft sunshine and whispering poplar leaves. What you are to me are what I saw myself as being and enjoying and loving. What you are to me is my day, my night, my breath and my being. What you are to me are the songs that are sung and the music that is made to move us. What you are to me fills me with so much joy that that is why I called you Joy, because it is what you fill me with. If you need to be reminded of your worth in the world and what someone thinks of you just say your name, Elona Joy. Beautiful Joy. The best kind. Know you are joy to me and your Nana Joyce and your father and your Nana Mimi.

If all mothers feel this way about their children, then this world is a wonderful place. This world is filled with love and promise and hope. Mothers fill the world with love for their children. This love fills the sky. If it were not for mothers and their love, then the world would be a lot less loving. For it begins here. Precious with precious. All six billion of us are loved. And that number is growing. Oh what a wonderful world!

My darling Elona. My little girl. You are my sky, my sun, my skin, my smile, my heart, mine. If this love of mine was harnessed, it would be the stars in the sky, the sun, the centre of the earth. Maybe it is? In the cosmic unlimitedness of living and life maybe it is. So if you look up at the stars and the sky and feel the ground you are surrounded by my love. You are held safely in love for all of your life for all of our love for all of our lives for all of us living.

24 April 2013

Great life, gnarl and nibble and nosh and gnash with incisors and broken bones and knives. Take this life, this ever-great life, this smarting, sensitized, quivering, vibrating, dazzling 82 years and wrap them round and stomp them down and smack them to and fro. Make them messy and loud and warm and above all full of love for her and you and me and us all. Bite big, bite hard, taste before you swallow, delight before you devour, dine with life in mind. Use your hands, use a fork, use bread, use *injera**, wrap it up in a tortilla, fry it over an open fire, boil it until the pot is black, burn it, bake it, fry it in hot frying fat so it sizzles, sear it in a smoking pan, adorn it with sprinkles, cover it in chocolate, smear it over toast, dip it, divide it, demolish it. I am five and all alive. I am five years and all alive. I am five years walked away from a bewildering day of topsy turnover life. I am five years and all awake. All alive.

I am grateful to myself for wanting to live and wanting to survive. I don't think I would be alive had I not wanted to live. Decisions made on whim, to check out a minor lump. I went because a small nagging voice said to go. I will listen to those small nagging voices from now on.

Do we have to talk of such grand things such as loving life and avoiding death and grieving? There are so many ungrand moments, so many banal days, so many complaints and dead leave days and broken dream moments and dirty dishes and disorganized drawers and mismatched socks and burnt roasts and worn out toothbrushes, and sticky fingerprints. Let me have these moments of wonder of pure pleasure and delight in living, in noticing the sun, of watching the slow unfurling of the leaves in spring, the moment before bursting is days away and the time in between is succulent and so lush full of lusty life. Tantalizing slow unrolling, minute by minute and day by day they unroll, but not until they are fully ready to unveil. They are enjoying these before moments. The before moments of the dessert spoon not yet on your tongue, your man's lips not yet touching yours but you can smell his smell, the time between the dive and the swim, the time between the strike of the match and the blaze, the time between the water drop and the ripple. We are all hushed and waiting for the unrolling of the leaves. The tree branches are heavier, holding the forthcoming unfurling. You can hear the water being heaved up from the ground in their tree veins to feed the mouths of leaves.

And you can tell me in any other moment that I'm not good enough and I might believe you. But in this moment, I am convinced of my divinity. I see my soul, so lovely and kind and gentle and forgiving and weak and questioning and childlike. I want to hold her, to love her. To raise her high in the air and rejoice at her goodness. I am a heartist – my heart wild and wide and smeared all over my body. My heart is on my sleeve, on my shirt, it is smeared all over my body. My heart is a wide open door. My heart is wide and full of holes and messy and embarrassing and if my gynecologist were here right now, I would make mad passionate love to him for being so kind and for bringing me the good news that I will go on.

Is it a relief? Why am I crying so much? Because I am so deeply happy to be me and to be me alive. The world without me. Space for something more cynical and deliberate, more directional. Space for commercial interests and manners and... what a weeping mass of mess.

I have curves and scars and I am not proud or defiant of these scars. I do not feel defiant. I would trade them back for the lack of experience, for no memory of pain, for no reminder of suffering, for no sense of the end. For the innocence of living invincibly. And what do I do with all these words? These piles of emotions, stacked, day over day. I don't want this day to end.

We lived in Belgium from June 2010 to July 2013. Kristof was working in Den Haag (The Hague, Netherlands), and commuting back and forth. I took care of Elona, learned Dutch, finished my PhD and tried to make my way in a new culture and language. We decided to move to Delft, (also in the Netherlands) in July 2013, so we could be closer to Kristof.

*Injera is a special bread made of fermented Teff flour. You use the bread to pick up and eat delicious Ethiopian food.

15 May 2015

Grief has a way of snapping you in the ass when you

didn't know it was lurking there. You can get cocky with grief, think you've slayed that beast. Grief is not a beast, it's just grief. And is that me talking or grief? If grief were talking, what would it say? Would it be angry? Grief is as complex as we are and you know it. You can feel its soft sadness, or a gulping, swallowing lump, or a wave of pain, or a white rage roar, or… you name it… I feel grief in my stomach. When my dad died, I could only lay down and cry, my stomach clenching and unclenching, holding and releasing sobs. It felt good and wise to sob for my love for him, to honour his place in my life. Why didn't I do that for myself? I didn't think I was worth grieving for… and yet I did, without acknowledging it, without speaking directly to it, I grieved. And many days I held it back, a wall around it, bricked it up, a stone wall surrounding it. Oh, the energy I took to hold it back. I was scared what they would think of me if I was sad all the time.

Really, I didn't know how to be with my cancer/pregnancy. I was a tragedy. Despondent, lost. Such a pit of self-pity. It was so ugly I couldn't stand to look at myself, be in myself. So many dreams twisted, torn and not what I thought it would look like. Newlywed life, research career, motherhood, breast-feeding. Thumping to the ground like dead birds. And then feeling guilty for feeling sorry for myself… that was it. I felt guilty for feeling sorry for myself. I was supposed to be feeling like a survivor. Geez. Really… I didn't feel like a survivor… I felt like I'd lost. Lost. Lost. Lost, loser. Loser. A big loser. And a big angry, ugly, lost loser who hated herself for feeling sorry for herself. Like I was supposed to be happy I had cancer while I was pregnant… why did I have this feeling? I had received the message from so long ago that I had to be quiet, be a good girl and put up with it… and smile. Smile.

So a repressed housewife I became. My fingers are releasing repression one word at a time. Gosh these are heavy words. They bear the weight of a life not lived my way. What I wanted. And because cancer had said to me… well… fuck you and your dreams… you're dealing with this… VICTIM. VICTIM. VICTIM I became. Oh, how terrible this feels… this VICTIM. Uh! She is even uglier than bald, unable to shit, fat-ass, cancer. She is smelly, unlovable, greasy hair, pimpled faced, well as ugly as an ugly woman can be. And no one loves an ugly woman. NO ONE. Not even me. And I am repelled by me the VICTIM. REPELLED. I can't stand her. Can't stand to be around her. Oh no… not her again. I don't want to hang around her.

VICTIM. It took me eight years to step aside from her. Years of learning, listening, pushing, I knew there was a way out... and I sought help. I asked, I paid for coaches to guide me. I did not do this alone. I am now comfortable hanging out with victims. It's like shadows of myself – that are still there if I turn away from the sun. And I recognize them and I'm not scared of them. Because I see I was a victim, playing – well, playing is far too much fun – being a victim, behaving, acting, thinking, snorting, living a victim's life. And I knew this just wasn't me.

22 September 2015

I had a checkup with the gynecologist. I still have my ovaries because I want a sex drive and by God, those ovaries are mine and I'd like to keep them.

I am screened for ovarian cancer. The doctor informed me that the protocols had changed. Screening is ineffective. One either had ovarian cancer or not. Makes sense. So my choice was chemotherapy or menopause. I don't mind menopause. But it makes me wonder, if they chop out all the parts that make me a woman, am I still a women? I guess my vagina, my brain, and years of social conditioning are what hold me in the space of womanhood. What does it mean when all the physical parts of being a woman are a danger to me?

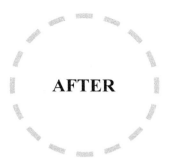

AFTER

In July 2015, I received my nipple tattoos from Alma Boerland (www.almaboerland.nl). A fantastic lady who specializes in making women feel beautiful. I invited filmmaker, and videographer, Susan Jimenez, to film the process. I had wanted to give myself a Nipple Party since I had my museum pieces created. The application of the tattoos signalled the end of rage. It was time for a party.

There were many moments when living was not a heroic act or a choice, just a day. Just a minute. Just a moment of nothing more monumental than breathing. I wanted to stand on top of myself, me the victim, the sad sack of self, the hero, warrior, failure, and say, "It's all right, you're okay. It's over." The pit of grief I wallowed in made a huge space to be filled and love rushed into that space. My Nipple Party was for me. For everyone. I wanted to encompass all of us into a moment of pleasure. A pinpoint of pleasure, just like my nipples. And I wanted everyone to join me in my joy.

Jasmina Campochiaro, a spiritual architect, was my project coordinator. She immediately saw why a Nipple Party was so important. She rushed around looking for funding, food and venues. Susan Jimenez created the Facebook page, the website and a documentary about my nipple tattoos. Hotel Vermeer in Delft provided the perfect venue.

Kim Brice, a somatic coach and Nia instructor, led us all in a Champagne Shimmy, which infused us with energy and joy. I invited everyone I knew – from former bosses, to long-lost family members, to colleagues, new friends and old friends. Everyone. My nipples were significant only to me before I had cancer. With My Nipple Party, they even have their own website, www.myNippleparty.com

Alma Boerland presented me with a photo of my nipple tattoo on chocolate. I immediately broke into an anticipation of nibbling on my own nipple!

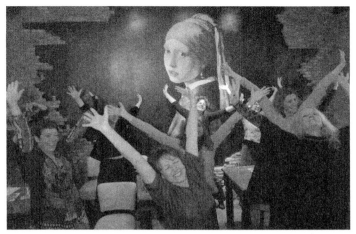

Photo 7: The Champagne Shimmy at My Nipple Party, Hotel Vermeer, Delft

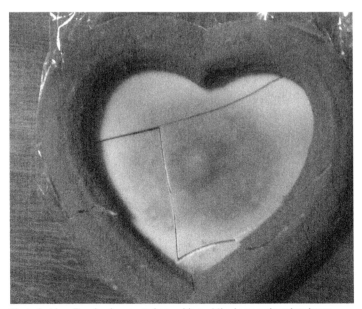

Photo 8: Alma Boerland presented me with my Nipple on a chocolate heart

My Nipple Party was celebrated on 25 October 2015. It was perfect. The room was full of love and people connecting with me and with each other. Alma Boerland talked about her work and showed us a video on how nipple tattoos are applied. Susan Jimenez made a documentary of Alma applying the tattoo to my chest. The documentary featured interviews with me and Kristof talking about our cancer. Seeing myself topless for the world to see was a 'gulp' moment. It is on my website www.suelawrence.co. To finish off the evening, Kim Brice led the room in Champagne Shimmy. We rocked our hips to booming music and yelled at the top of our lungs. It was a sensuous pleasure and a brilliant 'up' way to end the event. Throughout the evening friends came up to me and said, "Sue, you have to do more of this!"

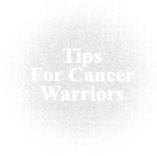

Tips
For Cancer
Warriors

DEALING WITH CHANGE

Once your treatment is done and your life does not revolve around doctors' appointments, you may notice a huge gulf where support used to be. Okay, you're done with treatment, now you can get back to being who you were before. Yet, you are not who you were before. At all.

My life, body, mind, soul were sent into a shredder and I stood there with the shards. I did not want to hear about other people's breast cancer stories and how they survived them. Nor did I want to suppress the fact that shit happened. Like any other trauma victim, I stood there agape at my monster body, through a fog of bewilderment, disappointment, sadness and totally lost. Who was I now? Who was that person, with the scars, stubby hair, the baby on her hip? I believe the time after cancer treatment is more difficult. The lack of attention was a shock. Not only was I terrified the cancer would come back, there was no one who understood what I was going through.

Find one person who gets the situation you're in. Marianne was mine. She wrote the Foreword for this book. She kept me sane all these years after cancer. It was a god-soaked coincidence that I met her in the recovery room after they pulled the needle out from my last chemotherapy.

GIVE TO YOURSELF FIRST

I only recently learned to give to myself first. Someone told me that the metaphysical aspect, the '*what is the message that breast cancer is sending me?*' is about giving so much of myself there is nothing left for me. If someone has said this to me during treatment, I would have smacked them up the side of the head. Do you mean I caused my own cancer?

I do accept that some dangerous recipe – comprised of a mix of biological, physical, psychological and spiritual elements – made my cancer. And I accept that, yes, I did give so much of myself there was nothing left for me. I put everyone else's needs before my own. My adrenal system, my body, my heart, myself – gave, gave, gave. And I didn't take care of me. Yet no one knows exactly what causes cancer. The scientists, with all their money and effort, don't know what causes cancer. How can I be so arrogant to think that *I* have the answer?

What I do know is that it was a horrible gift. It taught me many things. One is realizing that all those people I was straining to help were fine. They didn't need my help. Huh.

Yet giving makes me happy. The difference between the giving then and the giving now is that I give to myself first. I try to do this every day with writing, getting a good night's sleep, eating healthily, exercising and asking for help.

MARK MOMENTS

Mark moments that are important to you with a celebration or a moment of mourning. It acknowledges to yourself that you are important and this had an impact on you. Do something meaningful to you. Go on a trip. Light candles. Write a diary. Stay in bed and cry. Being ever the drama queen, I sent a photo of my cancerous breast down the Athabasca Falls, Jasper, Canada. Then, I had a Nipple Party complete with a documentary and a book. You don't have to go over the top like I did. Just make sure your important moments are not ignored by you.

4

TAKE YOUR TIME

Take your time with your cancer. People sped me through my cancer to the moment I would be a survivor when I had only just been diagnosed. Take the time to digest, grieve, decide, and recover. Healing also takes longer than you think – from diagnosis to treatment to recovery. Allow yourself plenty of time to rest and recover.

I was diagnosed with breast cancer in October 2007 during breast cancer awareness month. I hosted my Nipple Party October 25, 2015, eight years later. That's how long it took me.

RESPECT YOURSELF AND APPLY SELF-LOVE SALVE

Take yourself and your needs seriously. It's time to put *you* first. You know you've put everyone else's needs ahead of yours. Begin by becoming aware of what you do and what you say to yourself. Begin to nurture yourself and listen to what that tiny voice inside is saying. She's whispering something kind. Listen to her.

One of my sources of shame came from the financial burden I felt I was to my husband during my cancer treatment and recovery. I was draining the family finances because I was not earning an income, plus I was the only one spending (I bought all the food, clothes, and household items and paid the bills). Plus, I spent without thinking about the consequences. He and his family didn't overtly complain about my lack of income, yet it hung like a bad smell in the air during discussions over what I had spent money on. I defended myself by saying I was earning a PhD and building a baby and teaching part-time. Each time I tried to find a means to get out resulted in a further drain of our finances. Career coaching, book publishing, I was a drain – an open sewer for contempt to flow into.

Going through cancer and writing about it has shone the light in all my dark places. My self-talk was telling me I deserved no respect because I was not filling the bank. I even went so far as to say I was worth more dead because then my value would be seen. At the bottom of my soul was my voice saying, 'Mercy'. Through many years of support from coaches and daily writing, I whisper back to her lovely sweet things. I apply that self-love salve daily and liberally. I illuminate the dark places by shining some love and compassion on me. That light still goes out making me mean. In finishing this book, my perfectionist monster used her claws. I still have the scars.

GRIEVE

Grief goes along with change yet it deserves a point by itself. You may grieve all the changes. You are different and you will never be the same. Notice you're sad. Try to resist the urge NOT to feel pain. Kirsten Neff wrote a great book, *Self-Compassion: Stop Beating Yourself Up and Leave Insecurity Behind*. Her premise is that it is our resistance to pain that causes us to suffer. So suffer. It's painful. It's hard. It's a big deal, and it's a small deal. Just like my nipples.

How you grieve is very personal. I wrote and cried and complained. I beat myself up about crying and then I cried because I was beating myself up. (Self-love salve was applied here.) I wrote so much that it turned into a book.

How long you grieve is also very personal. I'm *still* grieving. In the process of preparing this book, I came across a photo we took of my breasts prior to all the surgeries. My little, imperfect breasts – I had hurled so much disgust at them. And now I'd do anything to have them back. And then this sad thought dissolves into the next, which is a little less sad until I surface back into the world of keeping busy. My breasts – a big deal and not a big deal.

FEAR

Hung in the wires of potential is hope and fear. Fear is about the future. What might happen? I swing between these wires. As I write this to you, I am preparing for another surgery. It's not life threatening but it's on my breast – the source of my sorrow – so I'm scared. I've set my intention (see point about Power and cancer below) and yet it's still there, this fear. I'm not frightened by my fear anymore. It used to paralyze me. I used to run away from it, distract myself with busy work in order NOT to feel fear. Now I greet its freeze with a nod and keep writing, which is my way of dealing with everything. Be aware of your fear. Wear it like a sweater, feel it in your body. Try to use it to move forward.

MARRIAGE AND RELATIONSHIPS

You may notice your cancer diagnosis will chase away those people who didn't really like you in the first place. It may push the buttons of those who love you. Friends will be awkward. Colleagues will pry. Family members will stand by with a worried look on their face in need of direction. Don't worry about them. Worry about you. You're the one who needs the care and attention. Take it. And maybe ask for help when you need it too.

Marriage is a different beast and I have no clear answers, because I only have my experience to draw on and that's far from perfect. Many marriages break down during breast cancer treatment. We had just gotten married. It seemed a little soon to get divorced. Bewildered by cancer and pregnancy, we stumbled forward. There were times when he didn't get why I was sad. I didn't understand why he didn't understand. I've just lost a body part, I'm being injected with poison and I'm carrying my child! How can you not get my pain?

Ah, Time. Distance. Denial. Humour. All wonderful tools we can draw on to get us through. Find your tool and try not to hit your partner over the head with it. One of my tools was to write.

Hot Sex

My husband, Kristof and I had hot sex last night. The bed moved a foot from the wall. The last time we had hot sex, my legs went up over my head in a backward somersault and I landed on my feet. We believe this manoeuver was the moment of conception of our daughter Elona.

I found a lump in my breast three months into the pregnancy, a month after we were married. Diagnosis – breast cancer. A dark blanket descended over my head. Our kisses went from gloopy and sloppy to dry and desperate. It was the end of hot sex for six years.

Newlywed bliss, pregnancy glow, were both erased by moving in with my mother and shuttling between doctor's appointments. Who I was depended on the day's appointment. Was I a young breast cancer patient – or an old pregnant lady? One day we were crying, the next filled with wonder at our growing baby. My husband, I barely saw him. I mean I was so focused on myself, the changes, the horror, guilt, fear, that I could not see him. I knew it was hard for him. He was living with his mother-in-law, far away from work and his family. His wife, his child, were in jeopardy.

I had a bowling-ball belly and a gash across my chest where my breast used to be. A span of skin was in its place. My heart was closer to the world now. My bald head sat atop it all and watched. The distance between myself and I was filled with grief and guilt. The distance between Kristof and I was uncountable.

Doctors said Elona would be safe with the chemotherapy. Our separate blood systems meant she wouldn't suffer. I was scheduled for six doses. Reddevil was the aptly named cancer drug given to breast cancer patients. A runny lava that burned as it infused my veins. It turned me weepy, my brain into soup, my eyes a river, my ass a tortured conduit.

Kristof was bewildered, but he remained constant. The same. I changed. My bloated, hairless body, a large white worm. A year later, the surgeon would say that he remembered my scruffy husband with the Belgian accent from when we met for the first breast removal. The surgeon did not remember me. Of course you don't remember me, I didn't say, I don't remember me.

Kristof and I went for counselling to try to keep afloat. The counsellor remarked how well we communicated, how close we were. Gosh, we gave a good show. We didn't speak about the horror, the guilt, the sorrow I felt as all my dreams for a nurturing pregnancy fell away with my hair. My deep joy with the idea of breast-feeding my child was chopped off. Kristof did not speak. He did not have these dreams. He had me and I was not me anymore. My husband said the drugs changed me and he missed his wife. I missed me too.

My hormones sustaining the pregnancy retreated and Elona was born six weeks early. Our little science experiment glowed blue under a plastic dome. I wanted to hold her but she had to lay protected from the world, with her eyes taped shut, tubes feeding her, monitors to make sure she breathed. Bald-headed, shame leaked from me, repelling nurses, doctors, myself. I had failed once again. I could not even keep this baby inside me long enough to make sure she received any good that was left in me. Three weeks later, we brought her home. Sleep deprivation and chemotherapy made my cognitive function close to a worm's. Kristof burst into fatherhood with relish. He was jubilant she was out of danger, out of my body. Fatherhood was something he could do something about. His wife's cancer, he was rendered useless. He didn't even know this woman anymore: her deformed, dried carcass, her mood swings.

I watched him hold her, nurture her, time her feeds with Excel spreadsheets. Oh, how I longed to be my child, to be held for hours, loved unconditionally. Motherhood did not come easy to me. Wifedom neither. Yet we carried on sustained by something, bigger than all of us, though I wasn't sure at the time what that was. We didn't kiss. My lips leather, his cracked from the dry winter weather.

After the pregnancy, I went on Tamoxifen, a medication that snuffed my hormones out in order to decrease the chances of cancer returning. For five years, this life saving drug stomped womanliness to the ground and left me feeling like a dull, burnt fuse, but I was alive. Grateful and busy with motherhood. Kristof was busy with work and spent swathes of time away from us. We acted like neighbours who shared a bed. Polite, doing our duties, remote. When we did kiss, it was dry and boring.

After a full five years, and with a doctor's nod, I stopped the medication. My periods returned in a flood. I became a woman again. I savoured every drop of blood, revelling in my curves, my temper, my desire for chocolate, my husband. After five years, we began to talk, and we talked, and we talked. Finally, we kissed. Strong, deep and hot.

MAINTAIN 'NORMAL' LIFE

Try to keep your foot in the door of your pre-cancer life, or a toe if that's all you can handle. Consider working with your employer to see how you can navigate your career through the storm.

Looking back now, I used a lot of energy to be normal when inside, I felt far from normal. And yet, I needed normal. I needed to know there was something else outside of this victimhood. There was a world that didn't deal with it minute by minute. I dove into my PhD because I understood how to be a PhD student. I was lucky I had a job teaching at the university via Distance Learning so I could work from bed. My colleagues didn't see my bald head and if they had pitiful looks, I couldn't see them.

POWER AND CANCER

Getting a diagnosis of cancer impacts your life. Fact. Navigating through doctors, treatment, post-treatment – it's a full-time, soul-draining job. The health professionals are there to take care of you to an extent. But it's you who has to make the hard decisions and endure their outcomes.

Prepare yourself by setting goals. Think about how you want appointments with your doctors to go. How do you want to feel during and after? Setting a goal such as, "I recover from my surgery with grace and strength" gives your energy a place to move towards. Make a choice to do some of your cancer with an infusion of power. You don't have to know how it's going to turn out. Just step forward with intention. Setting goals will help you to shift from self-pity to powerful in an instant. First, it takes awareness of self-pity. Then it takes a conscious decision to shift from self-pity to powerful. Believe me it takes practice.

I had a victim 'way of being' prior to cancer. I reeked of poor me. Cancer, chemotherapy, amplified this. After cancer, my husband suggested I get a coach to build my confidence. It took me (gulp) three years to recognize I was a pity party and a year more to yield my power for good.

My first deliberate shift from pity to powerful was during a visit with a Dutch oncologist. After five weeks of unexplained heavy bleeding, which I found disconcerting as I hadn't had a period for over a year, I went to a general practitioner. She made me feel as if my concerns were not important. Her look of bafflement at my stress sent me into the pity pit. She did, however, make me an appointment with an oncologist. Fed up with feeling a victim, I wanted something different from this appointment. One of my coaches at the time, Patty Walters, asked what I wanted to feel after this appointment. I wanted to not feel defeated. Not a victor either, not a warrior, just not defeated. I wanted a good clean fight where we both had our say. Patty is a big believer in play. She said, "Okay. How are you going to feel powerful?" She helped me come up with the pirate costume.

The appointment with the oncologist coincided with my daughter's school carnival and birthday party. She had chosen a pirate theme. I was a parent volunteer with the carnival and had to wear a costume. To kill two birds with one stone, I bought a pirate costume. Worked out in my head, it was carnival in the morning, oncologist appointment at lunchtime and birthday party in the afternoon. There was something about those over-the-knee boots, sword swinging, and pirate hat that put a swagger in my hips and filled me with power. My husband did not look at me once as we walked through the hospital.

I was clear, asked questions, breathed and was calm. I wanted the facts laid out on the table so I could make a decision. (Or I was going to cut her down with my sword.) This she did with respect and honesty. It was the BEST appointment I have ever had with a medical professional. It was only after our discussion that she asked, "Why are you wearing a pirate costume?"

FINDING JOY

Is it a coincidence that breast cancer hits us in middle age? I don't think so. I bet at the point of your diagnosis you were on the top of your game – juggling all the balls and feeling quite smug with your situation. And why not? You were doing it. It was all going so well.

A sledgehammer slammed into my life at the point where I was just taking off. It hurt. I had failed to reach any of my dreams. Yet, in the smoking ruins of my war, I found writing. Andrea Henning, one of my coaches, recommended Julia Cameron's *The Artist's Way: A Spiritual Path to Higher Creativity*. I began to write. A trickle, a flood, a book. I scramble to get to my writing pages every day. I plug into my joy every day. Find your joy. And do it every day.

HIRE GOOD HELP

I mention coaches a lot. I've worked with a lot of coaches during the past seven years. For me, they were better than friends because they were trained to keep their emotional baggage on their own conveyer belt as I swung around on mine. Plus, I'm paying them, so they'd better have it sorted out. I continue to work with a coach because they are the guide on the path ahead holding the light for me to follow. They are blessed friends. If you can't afford to pay for the coach of your dreams, check out their website. A savvy coach will have great, free resources to offer so you can taste their style of working.

GIVE THANKS

Marianne reminded me about this one. To give thanks. It sounds clichéd, but give thanks a little bit every day. It will help to keep things in perspective and lift your mood.

You're probably not surprised to hear this, but I'm an emotional person. My highs are wings and my lows are weights. Up until this morning, I felt ashamed for my emotions. Like I've soiled my underpants in public and everyone can smell me. In the summer of 2013, I started writing daily. I face myself on the page. Demons and doubts are hurled onto the page. After three pages I'm spent. From out of somewhere, a few sentences of thanks spurts out. Thanks for relieving me of my burden. Thanks for being. And in that moment, I am enough.

So now it's a daily habit to say "thank you". Thanks for this coffee, thanks for my family and friends, thanks for my Cancer…uh… sorry, not there yet…thanks for this life – this small one-in-six-billion of a life.

FINAL WORDS

Chemotherapy kills new cell growth, which means your body stops growing. Now, you get to grow again. In the direction you choose. What you do with your cancer is your choice.

Cancer showed me the edges of my life. It was my job to fill it in with practical actions and magic. And for various reasons, moving countries, having a baby, being on numbing Tamoxifen, I didn't. Instead, I fell into a pit of self-pity where I stayed. Writing this book was one of many actions which got me out of that pit. And I keep trying to get out of this pit. Day after day, I'll keep trying until I'm convinced of my silly magnificence. There is no one right way to be or do cancer. You have to be and do what you want to be with your cancer. It's your cancer.

RESOURCES

Listing all the breast cancer resources available here would not do them justice. If you're receiving treatment then hopefully the medical professionals will have suggestions.

I plan to write more about breast cancer so stay tuned via my website, www.suelawrence.co and Facebook page, My Nipple Party.

COACHES I'VE WORKED WITH:

Franciska Moor and **Andrea Henning** at Tiara Coaching International: http://tiaracoaching.com/Tiara
Marie Dewulf, Coach2MoveOn:
http://www.coach2moveon.com/wp/
Patty Walters at Rock Star Coaching: http://rockstar-business.weebly.com/about.html
Jan Stringer and **Alan Hickman** of Perfect Customers:
http://perfectcustomers.com/

BOOKS I'VE FOUND HELPFUL:

Brown, Brené, Ph.D., *Daring Greatly: How the Courage to Be Vulnerable Transforms the Way We Live, Love, Parent, and Lead*, Avery, 2015

Cameron, Julia, *The Artist's Way: A Spiritual Path to Higher Creativity*, Tracher/ Putnam, 2002

Cummings, e. e., *Selected Poems*, Liveright, 2007

Ephron, Nora, *I Feel Bad About My Neck: And Other Thoughts on Being a Woman*, Vintage, 2008

Lamott, Anne, *Bird by Bird: Some Instructions on Writing and Life*, Anchor Books, 1995

Lerner, Harriet, Ph.D., *The Dance of Anger: A Woman's Guide To Changing The Patterns Of Intimate Relationships*, W.M. Morrow, 2014

Lynch, Margaret, *Tapping into Wealth: How Emotional Freedom Techniques (EFT) Can Help You Clear the Path to Making More Money*, Tarcher, 2014

Milne, A. A., *The World of Pooh: The Complete Winnie-the-Pooh and The House at Pooh Corner*, Dutton Children's Books, 2010

Monk Kidd, Sue, *The Secret Life of Bees*, Penguin, 2003

Myss, Caroline, *Invisible Acts of Power: Channeling Grace in Your Everyday Life*, Atria Books, 2006

Neff, Kristin, *Self-Compassion:Stop Beating Yourself Up and Leave Insecurity Behind*, Harper Collins, 2011

Silverstein, Shel, *Where the Sidewalk Ends: Poems and Drawings*, Harper Collins, 2014

ABOUT THE AUTHOR

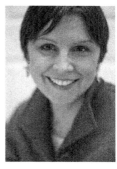 Sue Lawrence is a writer and researcher. She began her career as a community health nurse in Edmonton, Canada. Longing for adventure, she moved to the UK to earn her MPhil and study tobacco companies. She earned her PhD from Royal Holloway, London, UK, during her cancer treatment. Her study concerned risk and resilience factors to psychological disorder in high-risk Israeli youth.

She continues to work on this topic and is expanding trauma to include breast cancer. She has taught health policy via Distance Learning at the London School of Hygiene and Tropical Medicine for 11 years. She is the proud mother of Elona and the happy wife of Kristof. Running, exercising, cycling, travelling, building a community, and connecting with loved ones while eating great food are among her favourite things to do.

Sue would love to hear from you.

Please contact her at:
www.suelawrence.co
www.mynippleparty.com
https://www.facebook.com/itsyourcancer/?ref=hl

To buy copies of this book please contact Springtime Books at www.SpringtimeBooks.com

CPSIA information can be obtained
at www.ICGtesting.com
Printed in the USA
LVOW04s1915020916
502802LV00005B/15/P